T0067962

UNREVEALED REVELATION

A Remarkable Story of
Prostate-Cancer Survival

EDDIE CAPE

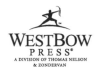

WESTBOW
PRESS®
A DIVISION OF THOMAS NELSON
& ZONDERVAN

WestBow Press books may be ordered through booksellers or by contacting:

WestBow Press
A Division of Thomas Nelson & Zondervan
1663 Liberty Drive
Bloomington, IN 47403
www.westbowpress.com
1 (866) 928-1240

ISBN: 978-1-9736-2102-7 (sc)
ISBN: 978-1-9736-2155-3 (e)

Library of Congress Control Number: 2018902386

Print information available on the last page.

WestBow Press rev. date: 03/27/2018

CONTENTS

PREFACE

With an internet search for "prostate cancer" yielding over five million responses, why would someone write a story on the subject, especially a layman with no medical background?

The purpose of my story is not to provide information about the disease, although some is included. It's to share how God directed me at a critical point in my prostate cancer battle to experiment with a nonmedicinal strategy. This test involved extensive research, hard work, discipline, minor lifestyle changes, a God-provided confidence to risk the unknown, faith (although weak at times), and a unique answer to prayer. It also involved responding to ideas that I would have never imagined and eventually learning how God remarkably provided all the equipment needed for my experiment. As you will read, the result was amazing!

This story targets three audiences, but it is fitting for others. First, it is to give hope to those who are struggling with nonterminal prostate cancer. Second, it is to encourage those of Christian faith who may be going through a physical valley in their lives. Third, it is to help bring those without faith to the warmth, peace, joy, and hope that Jesus Christ gives.

When God revealed to me how he had been working in the background for years—possibly decades—to make my disease turnaround possible, my excitement level rose to a point where I felt compelled and directed by the Holy Spirit to get this miraculous story distributed. There is nothing in my experience that cannot be used by most prostate cancer patients.

I must give special thanks to my beautiful wife of fifty years, who has been my rock and has given selfless support and encouragement to me throughout my illness. I would also like to thank all the medical professionals who have gone beyond their calls of duty while treating me. I would like to express my sincere gratitude to the Son's Creation Bible class and to the many people who have lifted me in their prayers. Special appreciation is given to my pastors, who have expressed their love, concern, and provided pastoral care to me during this time of uncertainty. Most of all, I want to thank my Lord and Savior, Jesus Christ, for comforting me and for providing divine guidance throughout this nine-year journey.

1

THE DIAGNOSIS

It was a cool evening in March 2008 when I received a call from my primary care physician. Earlier in the week, I had been in his office for a routine blood test associated with a diabetic condition. It was common for my good doctor to do other tests in addition to the one for diabetes. After giving me an acceptable A1C score, the tone of his deep, matter-of-fact voice changed to one of extreme seriousness. "Mr. Cape," he said, "your PSA is 8.7, and it should be less than 4.0. I want to do a second test in a month. A urologist may be in your future."

I had no idea at that time what a PSA test was or what a reading of 8.7 indicated. Due to the concern of my doctor, I could tell it was something serious and began doing research on the subject. I discovered that PSA is an abbreviation for prostate-specific antigen, a protein released by the prostate gland in men. Most PSA passes from the body, but some is passed to the blood. A PSA test determines the amount in the blood. If more than normal amounts are present, the prostate gland is likely, but not necessarily, diseased. It did not take long to realize that I could have prostate cancer, especially with a reading of 8.7.

Previously, my doctor was treating me with medications for BPH (benign prostatic hyperplasia), which is an enlarged prostate gland, for I had symptoms of one suffering from this condition: difficult and frequent urination. Other tests performed in his office indicated no unusual formations on my prostate gland other than enlargement.

My only previous firsthand experiences with prostate cancer were from my father and father-in-law; both had passed away from the disease. I recalled the mental and physical struggles my gentle and humble father had experienced twenty-eight years earlier when he was fighting the disease. I remembered the optimism he initially had when he began his treatments but how that optimism gradually waned as the disease grew progressively worse. I reflected over the unsuccessful and painful bone marrow transplant he had gone through; I thought about his determination to recover from a mild stroke he had while fighting the disease and driving him to the emergency room on two occasions when he was unable to urinate. I also remembered the expression of horror on the face of an apparently new prostate cancer patient when he saw the cancer-ravaged body of my father in the waiting room of a radiologist shortly before my father's death.

I have other recollections, but the most vivid was the last time I saw him alive. It was a beautiful, clear, Sunday afternoon in October, and God had begun to paint the leaves with rustic red on the dogwood trees in the yard of my parents' modest home. I entered the bedroom of my father and found him lying in the fetal position. It was in this position that his pain was most tolerable. He was semialert, in pain, heavily medicated, but not complaining. I'm not a sentimental person, but I felt strongly moved to tell him something that I had never shared with him as an adult—nor had he shared with me. It was something that I believed both of us knew about each other, for we had a good relationship. I simply said, "Daddy, I love you." Through his pain, he also said he loved me. After those words, he fell asleep, and I was never to speak with him again. Very early the following Wednesday morning, October 10, 1990, my mother called to tell me he was gone—two and a half years after being diagnosed with the disease. He was seventy-three.

I also reflected over the struggle my father-in-law had with his prostate cancer. His was much less aggressive than that of my father, having lived over twelve years after his was first diagnosed. He was under the care of the Veterans Administration, which provided to him the best treatments and medications available at the time. Both he and my father shared with me how their treatments were affecting their bodies, but I didn't fully understand at the time and did not do due diligence to find out.

My father-in-law was a self-motivated and independent man who continued to drive and do minor physical activities until one month before his passing. Advanced prostate cancer often attacks the bones. As he was getting up from a chair in his home, his left leg snapped below the knee. Due to bone deterioration, the break was impossible to set, so he was bedfast the last month of his life. One of the most difficult tasks I have done was to temporarily move him from his in-home hospital bed so it could have clean linens placed on it. It was not difficult due to his weight, for he was very frail at the time. The difficulty lay in knowing I was causing him excruciating pain as he was being moved. After the fracture, his condition failed rapidly and, at the age of seventy-eight, he was united with Jesus Christ in heaven.

As I learned more about this disease that affects one out of every seven men in the United States, thoughts and questions occupied much of my time. Would I experience the same fate and pain as my father and father-in-law? How long did I have to live? I was sixty-four at the time. Had medical science advanced to the point where the disease could be eradicated? What about my loving wife and three wonderful adult children? How many more years could I watch my grandson play basketball, and would I live to see him graduate from high school? Were my affairs in order? Was my personal faith in God strong enough to carry me through the possibilities that were potentially before me?

I naïvely hoped that a laboratory error was made while performing the initial PSA test. Needless to say this was a month of anxiety and personal reflection. It was a time to examine my spiritual condition, future, and values in life.

In mid-April, a second PSA test was done, and the result was not at all encouraging. My PSA was now 10.5, indicating a high probability that I did, in fact, have prostate cancer.

One method used to measure the aggressiveness of prostate cancer is the percentage change in one's PSA from one measuring period to the next. This rate of change is called velocity. In one month, mine had risen by 1.8 points, or 20 percent. At that rate, it would double in less than five months, an indication of aggressive cancer. My primary care doctor gave me some encouraging but reserved words about possible treatments and outcomes. He referred me to an experienced and well-respected local urologist who was also a urologic oncologist and surgeon.

I first met my urologist in May. I don't recall him performing a third PSA test, but he did a prostate exam. He, like my primary care doctor, felt no irregularities on my gland other than it being enlarged. Nevertheless, he definitely wanted to do a biopsy to determine exactly what was going on.

Within two weeks, the biopsy was completed, and results were in. The biopsy itself was not too painful. I lay on my left side on the procedure table while the doctor took twelve samples. There was a slight sensation of pain each time, but the pain immediately subsided.

As fearfully anticipated, the biopsy indicated prostate cancer on the left side of my prostate gland.

My urologist gave me three treatment options, but I added a fourth. Option one (the one not mentioned by my doctor) was to do nothing until I had additional symptoms. After a bit more research and thought, this option was quickly dismissed. Once symptoms occurred beyond those already present, the possibility of long-term eradication and survival was greatly diminished, if not impossible. The three recommended by my urologist seemed plausible. They were radiation, removal of the prostate gland (prostatectomy) with an open incision, or a robotic prostatectomy.

It was discovered that radiation and both types of surgery would, essentially, yield the same outcome. If life expectancy of the patient was more than ten years, some professionals believed that a prostatectomy would be the best option. If life expectancy was ten years or less, the same experts recommended radiation. However, there appeared to be no real consensus among urologists over which was best.

The least invasive and least painful of the three was to have radiation therapy, called brachytherapy. With this, radioactive seeds would be placed in the prostate gland, possibly followed by seven weeks of external beam radiation. Having multiple radio-active seeds placed in an already enlarged prostate gland would, logically, make the gland even larger. The larger gland would, therefore, make it more difficult to void since it would compress the urethra, which goes through the walnut-size prostate gland. It is unknown if my reasoning was correct; I didn't ask. This condition would last until the cancer was killed and the size of the gland was diminished. In addition, there would likely be the seven weeks of daily radiation therapy. It was also my fear that some cancerous cells might be missed with radiation. For these reasons, a prostatectomy was my chosen option, but would it be open surgery or robotic?

An open-incision prostatectomy was considered but not selected. My urologist was an experienced and skilled surgeon in performing this procedure, but the hospital stay would be several days, and a fairly large incision would have to heal. Open incision was ruled out simply because I did not want to spend several days in the hospital and then go home with a large wound that would have to heal. In retrospect, I should have given this option more consideration.

The third was to have a robotic radical prostatectomy. This type of surgery was an outpatient procedure for which I would stay overnight in an outpatient hospital room and go home the day following surgery. There would be no large incision and recovery would be faster.

After making the decision for a robotic prostatectomy, my urologist, untrained in robotic surgery, gave me the name of another well-known and experienced surgeon who was a member of the same group of urologists as he. Based on information I could obtain, this doctor had performed over one thousand robotic prostatectomies and was the local go-to person for this type of procedure. (At the time, robotic surgery was a relatively new procedure for prostatectomies with few locally trained surgeons.) I called and made an appointment with him, but, as I recall, the earliest he could see me was in July. While making this appointment, I also learned that his fee was several thousand dollars and that he did not accept insurance. This was a financial red flag to me—not that he was unprofessional, dishonest, or greedy, but that I did not want to spend money unnecessarily if other options were available.

Finally, after fretting for several weeks over the thought of paying this fee when I had good insurance, a small inward voice gently told me to look for another doctor. I did and discovered there was a second professional in this group who was also a very experienced urologic surgeon and who was trained in performing robotic prostatectomies. However, instead of having done over one thousand robotically, he had done only sixty-four. I made an appointment with the less experienced doctor and canceled with the other. I met with him in early August, and the procedure was scheduled.

2

TREATMENTS

PROSTATECTOMY

On September 2, 2008, I checked in the hospital and was in a small holding room with my comforting wife awaiting surgery. My pastor arrived, spent some time with us, said some encouraging words, had prayer, and left. I was at peace, had no anxiety, and was excited over having this cancerous beast removed from my body.

Around 1:00 p.m., I was rolled into the operating room. I had never had surgery before. The room was what I thought it would be—several people wearing their surgical smocks and head coverings. The room was brightly lit and sterile-looking; a light was above me where I was placed for surgery. To my left was what I believed to be the DaVinci robot. It was a pedestal-looking device equipped with several pivoting and hinged arms surrounding and attached to it. It appeared to be approximately five to six feet tall, was blue, and looked something like one might expect to see in a NASA space device. It is difficult to provide a better description because from the time I entered the operating room until I was asleep was very brief—probably less than three minutes. I was greeted by the anesthesiologist, who stated his name and said he was going to put me to sleep. That is the last I remember until I was in the recovery room. In fact, the only thing I recall in the recovery room was a nurse saying, "Mr. Cape, wake up; your surgery is over."

I vaguely remember being rolled to my outpatient room where I would spend the next twenty hours. As I became more alert, I soon realized that I was connected to several types of monitoring devices and an IV, but my greatest memory was the catheter, a new experience for me.

I had very little pain; perhaps I was pumped full of painkillers. As the afternoon progressed and evening came, I became quite uncomfortable—not from surgical pain but from lying in the hospital bed in an awkward position. I was delighted when the attending nurse came and took me for a stroll through the hallway in my hospital gown and gold rubber-stripped nonslip socks. As I walked, the reservoir for my IV was attached to a small rack that I pushed, which was equipped with casters. My catheter holding bottle was strapped to my leg. I now had minor pain and soreness in my pelvic area.

When nighttime came, I easily fell asleep but was awakened several times during the night by my nurse who checked my vitals. I do remember being extremely thirsty at one point, around 2:00 a.m. My caring wife was asleep in a reclining chair near my bed, but the tray that held the water was out of my reach. She was sleeping so well, I did not want to awaken her. I finally went back to sleep until around 4:00a.m., when the nurse came in and said it was time for another walk.

After the walk and as I settled back in my bed, my nurse asked a question that totally surprised my wife as well as me. She asked, "You are Christians, aren't you?" We responded that we were. We then talked a few minutes about our faith. How she knew we were Christians, I have no idea, for we had made no verbal testimony to her nor had we even made any mention of our church or Savior, Jesus Christ.

The following morning, I was notified that I would be released later that day. The surgeon did not come to my room but left instructions, which were relayed to me by a nurse. One instruction was to make a one-week follow-up appointment with my surgeon, which was done. At that appointment, the catheter would be removed, and results of the procedure would be given.

Very little was known about my condition when I was released other than the surgeon telling my wife earlier that he had removed a "very large" prostate gland.

There was a small one-and-a-half-inch incision in my abdomen where the gland was physically taken from my body. In addition, three or four Band-Aid-size cuts were in my stomach area; I was now sore throughout my lower abdomen. At checkout, I was rolled to the car in a wheelchair but got in the car with no assistance. At home, I exited the car on my own and was glad to have that chapter of my life behind me.

The catheter remained and was inconvenient and slightly uncomfortable, but tolerable.

One week later my wife and I were in the surgeon's

waiting room. After a few minutes, we were called to meet with him. He asked a few questions to ensure that I was healing properly and then proceeded to review with us the pathology report. Although much of the information he provided was not comprehended, I did understand the cancer had positive margins; he was unsure if all the cancer cells had been removed. There was a possibility the cancer had spread beyond the gland, although he only hinted at that possibility and did not directly say so. His work was essentially complete, and he suggested that I could continue under his care or return to my original urologist, if I wished. The decision was made to return to my original urologist since his office was much closer to my home.

The next order of business that morning was to have the catheter removed. His nurse had previously instructed me to bring a pad, which I did—a small female variety that my wife had on hand. I went to another room where a nurse removed the catheter. Was I surprised! I realized immediately that I was totally incontinent and put on that small pad, which was grossly inadequate for the job at hand. Nevertheless, I made the best of it and was very happy that I did not have to get out of the car before arriving home.

It is common for men who have prostatectomies to experience incontinence. Men have two muscles that control their urination—an internal and external sphincter (muscle). The internal sphincter is inside the prostate and is removed when the gland is removed, leaving the external to control urination. During surgery, the external sphincter may be slightly damaged or may be weak, preventing it from functioning properly. The result is partial, and sometimes total, incontinence, which usually goes away after several days, weeks, or months. The recommended remedy for this condition is Kegel exercises, which aid in building the muscle. Although I did the exercises as suggested, this problem did not improve at all for several months. Finally, I did void naturally six months after surgery, but the volume was very light. From that point forward, this condition improved, and I was experiencing nothing but stress incontinence within a year. Stress incontinence is leakage when lifting heavy objects or when sneezing or coughing.

After surgery, I was given instructions to refrain from heavy lifting and doing strenuous manual labor for five weeks.

Three weeks after surgery, I felt good physically. The soreness was gone, and the small incision was healing nicely. I did have a UTI at one point, but that was easily eradicated with a prescription of antibiotics. Mentally, I was at peace, for I knew I was under the care of the great physician, Jesus Christ. However, I did have doubts about my future due to the pathology report, which I had reviewed, researched, and analyzed the best I could.

On the pathology report were several items that described the extent of my condition. First was the *Gleason* score, a numerical measurement between 2 and 10 that rates the aggressiveness of prostate cancer. It measures cancerous cells against good cells. If there is little difference, cancerous cells are assigned a low score of 1. If they are moderately different, they are graded 2 through 4, and if they are highly different or abnormal, they are assigned a score of 5. Apparently, there are two grades of cancer cells in a sample—those most common and those less common. First, the most common are evaluated and assigned a value. Second, the less common are analyzed and also assigned a number. The sum of the two numbers is the Gleason score, with 2 being the lowest possible and 10 being the highest. For example, samples measuring 3+3 would have a Gleason score of 6. A score of 6 or less indicates cancer that is likely to spread less aggressively than one with a higher reading. A score of 7 indicates a moderately aggressive cancer, while a score of 8 through 10 indicates a tumor that is highly aggressive. Mine was 4+3, or 7, indicating that I had moderately aggressive prostate cancer. A score of 7 with sample results of 3+4 is less aggressive than one with 4+3.

A second item on the pathology report was *perineural invasion* (PNI). PNI was detected, which meant that cancer was found along a nerve that penetrated the prostate gland. This nerve, in turn, could carry cancerous cells outside the gland into surrounding tissue.

A third significant item on the report was *stage,* a designation to determine how advanced the cancer was. Understanding staging is a little tricky and involved. The staging of prostate cancer uses a TNM designation. The T, followed by a number from 1 through 4, represents how far the cancer has spread; the N represents lymph-node invasion, and the M is a designation that represents whether the cancer has metastasized.

T1 tumors are confined to the prostate gland and cannot be felt during examination. In this stage, cancer is found either by a rising or elevated PSA reading or, more accurately, from a biopsy.

T2 tumors are also confined to the prostate gland and can be felt by examination and/or an elevated PSA. A prostate gland has two lobes. If the tumor is in less than half of one lobe, it is designated as T2a; if it is in more than half of one lobe, it is staged as T2b. Finally, if it is designated as T2c, the tumor is in both lobes.

T3 tumors have spread beyond the prostate gland to surrounding tissue and may be present in the seminal vesicles. If the pathology report stages the cancer as T3a, it has spread outside the gland. If it is T3b, the tumor is also in the seminal vesicles.

T4 tumors have spread beyond the gland to organs such as the rectum, bladder, external sphincter, or the pelvic area. T4 prostate cancer is sometimes graded as D1 or D2. With D1, the cancer still remains in the pelvic area, but with D2 it has metastasized to other parts of the body and may be in the bones.

The N portion of the TNM staging method determines if cancer is in the lymph nodes. An NX designation means that the lymph nodes were not tested, whereas an N0 (i.e., zero) means that no cancer cells were found in the tested pelvic lymph nodes. An N1 designation means that cancer was found in the lymph nodes.

Finally, M designates spread of the cancer, or metastasis.

M0 (zero): Cancer has not spread beyond nearby lymph nodes.

M1: Cancer has spread outside the pelvic area.

M1a: Cancer has spread to lymph nodes beyond the pelvic area.

M1b: Cancer is in the bones.

M1c: Cancer is in other parts of the body.

Staging on my pathology report was T3a, NX, MX, which meant that my tumor had spread beyond the prostate gland to surrounding tissue and that lymph nodes and metastasis were not checked.

Prostate cancer patients who are facing prostatectomies may wish to ask their surgeons if they do nerve-sparing surgery. There are nerves attached to the prostate gland that control the ability of men to have erections. With a prostatectomy, these nerves have to be carefully separated from the prostate gland. The delicacy of this procedure has been compared to separating wet tissue paper from a balloon. In almost all prostatectomies, there is some damage done to these nerves, which renders the patient impotent for a period of time. After several months (usually less than twenty-four) these nerves heal, restoring natural functionality. If, however, the surgeon is unable to separate the nerves successfully or if cancer is found in them, they are not spared, and the patient no longer has the ability to perform, even with medication. More details concerning this issue may be obtained online by searching for "nerve-sparing prostatectomies." There are nonsurgical and surgical solutions to this issue explained elsewhere.

My first PSA test after surgery was two months later, on November 10, 2008. It was done by my regular urologist, and the results were very encouraging. The PSA reading was undetectable. The next test was March 5, 2009, and measured .11, not overwhelmingly alarming but alarming enough to show that the disease was still present. After a prostatectomy, one's PSA should either be undetectable or close to undetectable and should remain at that level. An increase indicates that the disease is still present. By June

2009, my PSA was still increasing, and a joint decision was made between my urologist and me to radiate the prostate bed. It was hoped the removed tumor had not spread beyond that point, and if that hope proved to be true, radiation would kill the remaining infected cells. I was referred to a radiologist.

RADIATION THERAPY

The first appointment with the radiologist was in August 2009. After answering several written pages of very personal questions in his waiting room, I was called to his office where my case history and responses to the questions were reviewed. I was advised that I would receive over seven weeks of radiation—a total of thirty-eight sessions. Next, I was sent to the radiation room, where two technicians took various measurements of my body, marked it, and gave me two tiny tattoos, one on each leg on the outside of each thigh. I was told the tattoos would be permanent but were necessary. I assume they would be used to align the radiation machine. They were about the size of the head of a pin.

The following week I began radiation treatments. They involved lying on my back in a fixed position while the technician operated the radiation machine from an adjoining control room. While being radiated, I could not move lest the radiation beams hit the wrong target. The radiation machine rotated around my body, sending beams to the prostate bed from multiple angles. As the machine rotated, it was stopped several times. I assume radiation was given when the machine stopped. Each treatment lasted around ten to fifteen minutes.

While some people have side effects from radiation, I had almost none. The only side effect I experienced was minor fatigue. I'm unsure if it was from the radiation or the daily routine of driving in heavy traffic for the therapy. A registered nurse acquaintance said it could have been due to stress on the body while trying to heal itself from radiation. Whatever the cause, it went away a few days after treatment.

I was pleased to have that treatment behind me and waited anxiously for my first PSA test result, which did not come until the following April 2010, and it was .15. Six months later, in October 2010, it had become apparent that the radiation therapy had not worked and that the cancer had likely spread beyond the prostate cavity. My PSA was now .23. This is a very low reading, but it had increased significantly, over 50 percent, from my April reading.

The next agreed-to strategy between my radiologist, urologist, and me was to watch and wait until my PSA reached 5.0. At that point, I would begin androgen deprivation therapy (ADT). After prostate removal and radiation therapy, ADT was the next line of defense for me.

ADT is, essentially, a medicinal orchiectomy. Prostate cancer feeds off the male hormone, androgen, and by it being suppressed, prostate cancer progression frequently goes into remission for an unspecified period of time. It varies among patients. In simple terms, there are two types of ADT. One prevents the body from making androgen, and the second blocks androgen from being absorbed by cancerous cells. If cancerous cells are not fed, they die. My urologist informed me that he had patients who had been on it for eleven years and were doing fine.

An issue with ADT is its possible side effects. These include such things as hot flashes, cognitive degradation, lack of desire and ability to be sexually intimate, fatigue, weight gain, loss of muscle mass, and several others. None of these appealed to me.

The strategy I had selected for administering ADT, if it came to fruition, was intermittent therapy. With this method, treatment is administered until the patient's PSA drops to a very low level, at which time it is temporarily suspended. ADT resumes when the PSA again rises to a predetermined level. The advantage of intermittent therapy is that it offers a temporary break from side effects. Because intermittent ADT is a fairly new strategy, there is inadequate history to determine how it may impact the survival of the patient.

Another issue with ADT, whether regular or intermittent, is that eventually it loses its effectiveness. The body of the patient becomes refractory, or unresponsive, to the treatment. At that time, PSA will increase.

The watch and wait strategy remained in effect until September 2013—three years after the decision was reached to use ADT when my PSA reached 5.0. At that time my PSA had increased to 3.43. My urologist offered a possibility that could potentially help him with my treatment. He suggested that I go to the Mayo Clinic in Rochester, Minnesota, and have a C-11 Choline PET scan.

C-11 CHOLINE PET SCAN

An issue with advanced prostate cancer is the inability to determine where in one's body the cancer is until it is sometimes too late. The patient may be free from symptoms and feel great while the cancer is active and growing. By the time it progresses enough to be detected with a normal MRI or becomes symptomatic, such as bone pain, it may be too advanced to treat successfully. A patient's PSA may be increasing and have a high reading, but the location(s) of the cancer cannot be found. If the site of the cancer can be determined soon enough, it can, potentially, be locally treated.

To address this dilemma, a test is administered by the Mayo Clinic in Rochester, Minnesota, called the C-11 Choline PET scan. At this writing, it is believed no other organization in the United States is FDA approved to perform this test. Other tests are being developed, but this is the only one known at this writing that can determine the location of nonsymptomatic prostate cancer more accurately than an MRI.

The test involves inserting C-11 Choline in the bloodstream, which attaches to the cancer. The body is scanned. If cancer is detected, it will be highlighted when images of the scan are read. Although this test may not be 100 percent accurate, it is better than anything else now available.

Fortunately, an appointment was quickly arranged for me at the Mayo Clinic with assistance from my urologist. On Wednesday, October 2, 2013, I was at the clinic processing the necessary paperwork. The following day, Thursday, I had two tests—an MRI in the morning, and the C-11 Choline test in the afternoon. On Friday morning I met with a doctor from the urology staff at the clinic for feedback. This professional was instrumental in developing the test and getting it approved by the FDA. Test results showed four cancerous lymph nodes in the pelvic area.

While in the doctor's office, my local urologist was telephoned, and the two discussed test results and the clinic's treatment recommendations. I quietly listened on the speakerphone while the two discussed my case. Although I had no idea what their technical terminology meant, I did clearly understand two things: cancer was in four of my pelvic lymph nodes and surgical removal, followed by ADT, was the recommended treatment plan. I was not ecstatic over the test results or the proposed solution, but I was thankful the cancer was found and could be removed.

My wife and I are from the Atlanta area and live in a nearby town. Although the trip to the Mayo Clinic was over 1,100 miles from our home, we decided to drive. After our purpose at the Mayo Clinic was finished, our plan was to drive further north and take a minivacation in Bemidji, Minnesota. One of our destination points was Itasca State Park, where the Mississippi River begins.

My career before retiring, occasionally, took me to Minnesota, Wisconsin, and Illinois, but my business was always in Minneapolis, Madison, and Chicago. I flew into each city, conducted my business, and flew out. I had never actually seen the Midwest countryside. I was overwhelmed to witness the massive alfalfa and cornfields and flat land; they were breathtaking. It did not take me long to understand why a friend from the Midwest laughs at the cornfields we have in north Georgia. Also, I had no idea so many power-generating windmills were in use.

We especially enjoyed the lovely drive from Rochester to Bemidji. Massive grainfields were replaced with gently rolling hills, trees, crystal-clear lakes, forests, and beautiful farms.

Our day at Itasca State Park was notably memorable. It was early October, and the hardwood tree leaves were a gleaming gold, often forming a canopy over the beautiful drive through the park. As the sun reflected off their foliage, the trees were illuminated with a blinding brilliance. Lake Itasca was unusually attractive that day as we relaxed in the lodge while overlooking its clear, blue water. There was a cool autumn breeze, causing small whitecaps to form on the lake.

As I reflected over the diverse beauty of God's creation, it reminded me of His almighty power, and I was comforted, even though my earthly future was uncertain.

God reveals his physical secrets to humankind, who uses this information for earthly advancement and, unfortunately, occasional regression. Regardless of how impressive the discoveries and developments of humanity can be, they are dwarfed by God's life-sustaining and beautiful handiwork, power, sovereignty, and love.

Back home, I had been warned beforehand by the Mayo Clinic that my insurance would likely not cover the cost of the C-11 Choline PET scan, which proved to be true. It did, however, pay its share of everything else that was done, such as the MRI, blood tests, and so forth. For several months I received a bill for the test, amounting to thousands of dollars. Each bill said to not pay because the insurance claim was pending. Finally, after eight or nine months, I received a statement that showed zero balance. The Mayo Clinic knew the insurance would likely not pay, and I knew it wouldn't, and I was prepared to write a check for the test. After inquiring about the zero balance, I was astonished to learn that the clinic absorbed the amount due, and I owed nothing. What a pleasant surprise and gift!

LYMPHADENECTOMY

The next order of business in this cancerous adventure was to make the necessary arrangements through my surgeon-urologist to have the involved lymph nodes removed. On October 30, 2013, I checked into the hospital to have this procedure. Unlike the robotic prostatectomy, this was open surgery, resulting in a five-inch vertical incision in my lower abdomen and a three-night stay in the hospital.

The day following surgery, my doctor checked on me in the hospital room and gave some feedback. Instead of removing four lymph nodes, he had removed thirty-five, all in my pelvic area. I reasoned from his conversation that he was not comfortable with the surgery results. The statement that stuck with me was his comment that he hoped the surgery had not been done in vain. To me, this was an indication that something serious was going on. I was to see him one week later in his office.

The week between surgery and my appointment was not the best of my life. Even though I could sense that the biopsy results would probably be disappointing, I was at peace over the whole cancer situation. God was comforting me emotionally; other people seemed to be more concerned than I. What was unpleasant was the fact that my body did not like or appreciate at all having surgical staples in it! The incision did not hurt very much, but the places where the staples penetrated my skin were the points of pain. The area became badly inflamed and hurt constantly, even with pain medication. To be a bit more comfortable, I wore suspenders instead of a belt. After several weeks, the incision had sufficiently healed to pitch the suspenders.

At the one-week appointment, the staples were removed, and it was learned that nine of the thirty-five lymph nodes were cancerous. The biopsy stated that one was almost completely involved, an area of "extracapsular lymph node extension" was seen on five, and an "area of soft tissue metastasis was seen associated with lymphovascular invasion" on another. Two were labeled as having the presence of "metastatic carcinoma." The remaining twenty-six had no cancer. I was unsure exactly what those terms meant other than there was metastasis present, and cancer might be present in surrounding tissue in certain places. The watch and wait strategy was once again implemented.

My first PSA test after the lymphadenectomy was hopeful. It was taken in December 2013, and was 1.48, down from 3.43 prior to surgery. However, by April 2014, it had again climbed to 2.73, a dangerous increase of 84 percent. At this rate of increase, I would almost reach the 5.0 ADT threshold by my next test, scheduled for the following August.

CHRISTIAN FAITH

For a Christian, death is a promotion. In simple terms, it is the time when a person's soul (i.e., one's eternal immaterial essence) is separated from his or her physical body on earth and is connected with a new resurrected body in heaven. There are different theological chains of thought from Bible scholars concerning what happens to the soul of a Christian between death and this new life. One belief is that the person is judged and is then immediately united with a resurrected body in heaven. Another thought is that the soul's destiny (heaven or hell) is immediately determined at physical death but then temporarily resides in a holding place until Christ returns, when it then goes to heaven. Another thought is that the soul dies with the body and remains "asleep" until Christ returns, at which time it is resurrected with a heavenly body. There are others, but the bottom line is that those who have repented and have been forgiven of their sins, who have surrendered their lives to the resurrected Jesus Christ, who have accepted Him as their personal Savior, and who have adhered to the teachings of Christ by living a holy life will be saved from eternal punishment and rewarded with a new and permanent life in a place called heaven. The debate concerning what happens to one's soul between physical death and heaven will likely continue until Christ Himself returns.

The anticipation of this eternal paradise gives Christians an optimistic hope and positive attitude that many others do not enjoy. Even with the promise of eternal life in heaven, almost all people, Christians or not, instinctively want to live a mortal life as long as possible and will do whatever it takes to keep themselves alive. At some point, however, everyone must go through the valley of physical death.

Medical science is amazing and has made remarkable advances over the years. Eradication or near elimination of certain diseases such as smallpox and polio, control of life-threatening disorders such as diabetes, drug therapies for cancer, organ transplants, and many other advances can all be attributed to medical research and development. Therefore, I am an advocate of this science and its application. It is a wonderful contribution to humanity.

One could view medicine as the combined use of God's created elements and acquired human knowledge, technology, and skill to modify or stop the natural progression of an illness or injury. Application of medicine, medical procedures, and technology may stop or curtail the destruction of a disease or enable an injury to heal. Vast resources are spent each year to discover the causes and cures for diseases such as cancer.

There are times when medicine fails, does not have a solution, or reaches its known limits. At those times, many begin to rely on their faith and ask God to intervene. It is unfortunate that some call on God as their last resort instead of their first. God, through His loving mercy, often provides comfort, peace, and assurance to those who seek Him in periods of illness and uncertainty. Those who fail to rely on God during these times may miss the warmth that only Jesus can give. Psalm 55:22 reinforces the notion that God cares for His people: "Cast your cares on the Lord, and he will sustain you; he will never permit the righteous to be shaken." If the ailing do not cast their cares on the Lord, they may carry their burdens alone.

When one calls on God for healing, He may answer the petition as requested, He may answer differently than asked, or He may even respond with a no. Regardless of how God answers, the Christian believer knows that God is in charge and that He promises to be with His followers through life's most difficult circumstances, even grave illnesses.

Some people misunderstand and even misuse prayer. The purpose of prayer is not to try to persuade God to conform to the will of the one praying, but for the petitioner to seek and discover the will of God for the circumstance over which he or she is praying. With this attitude of prayer, we are essentially asking God to show us how to go through our circumstance. We may ask Him to remove our situation, but He may instead respond by providing direction concerning how to go through it. We place our confidence and trust in Him when navigating life's difficult roads. "Trust in the Lord with all your heart and lean not on your own understanding; in all your ways submit to him, and he will make your paths straight" (Proverbs 3:5–6). By going through our difficulties, our faith becomes stronger and we are better equipped to serve God.

When one petitions the Lord, he or she has faith, or confidence and trust, that the request can and will be answered. In the Bible, 1 John 5:15 reads, "And if we know that he hears us—whatever we ask—we know that we have what we asked of him."

One understanding of the above verse is that John is referring only to spiritual matters. A second and broader interpretation is that "whatever" refers to anything that is not against the will and purpose of God. If one accepts the second meaning, it would certainly include a physical illness.

Moreover, if the second interpretation is believed, it should not be taken to be a Santa Claus promise. Instead, part of Christian faith is the acknowledgment and understanding that prayers of all types, including those for healing, are answered according to God's purpose and plan. They are not always answered in such a way to make an individual feel physically better, although God is merciful and frequently responds that way.

From a human perspective, the ability to understand and accept disappointing answers from God is often difficult. The Christian believer looks toward heaven in these types of situations and relies on scriptures such as Romans 8:28: "And we know that in all things God works for the good of those who love him, who have been called according to his purpose." We may never understand some of God's answers, but we can certainly accept them. When they are accepted, life becomes easier. We can then plan and live around His answer, knowing that we are in compliance with His desire for us. When God failed to answer the apostle Paul's three-time request for the removal of his "thorn," he accepted God's answer and used it to his spiritual and missional advantage (2 Corinthians 12:1–10).

Another part of Christian faith is action. This principle is clearly stated in the Bible in the book of James: "Faith by itself, if it is not accompanied by action, is dead" (James 2:17). I once knew a lady who was diagnosed with breast cancer but refused to seek medical treatment. I believe this lady said a good-faith prayer for healing, but within one year she was deceased. Had she pursued the action of getting medical treatment, she possibly could have been healed through medical science. There, apparently, was no intervention from humankind or God, and the lady succumbed to her illness. Although her faith was strong, her actions were weak. God didn't kill this lady by not answering her prayer as petitioned; instead, He answered by allowing the disease to take its natural course.

At one point during my illness (between radiation treatments and lymphadenectomy), my good pastor asked if I would like to be anointed with oil and have him offer a prayer of healing on my behalf. I agreed and was anointed and prayed for in a public worship service one Sunday morning. I had faith that God could immediately heal but, I must confess, my personal prayer was different from that of my pastor. My prayer was that God's will be done over the whole matter and for Him to continue to give me peace.

There are different understandings among Bible scholars regarding the interpretation of certain scriptures referring to anointing with oil for physical healing. Both James 5:14 and Mark 6:13 seem to support the practice. James states, "Is anyone among you sick? Let them call the elders of the church to pray over them and anoint them with oil in the name of the Lord." The scripture in Mark says, "They [i.e., the disciples] drove out many demons and anointed many sick people with oil and healed them." Some interpret the "sick" in these verses to be those who are spiritually rather than physically ill. Others understand physical healing to be a practice used by Christ to authenticate his Messiahship – a ritual that was only applicable during His incarnation. Regardless of the interpretation, the Creator of the universe and the God I worship certainly has the power to heal the physically ill if He chooses.

After that service, there was no improvement in my

condition. My PSA continued to rise, and I continued to seek medical help. God did then and continues now to answer my prayer for peace. He has enabled me to dwell on things other than my illness.

During this same time my loving wife left each morning on the bathroom vanity where I do my morning routine a positive promise from the Bible. These handwritten verses gave me encouragement for the day and reminded me that a power much greater than humanity was in charge. She did this for over a month.

3

VITICULTURE

Several years prior to learning I had prostate cancer, I had a notion to plant a small vineyard. I can't explain why or how this idea came to me. I don't drink wine and have no idea how to make it. I enjoy grape juice, but not as much as other juices. If I wanted to, I could easily get enough grapes to make homemade jelly for my needs from a local produce stand, the supermarket, or a pick-your-own vineyard. Sometimes, discount stores in my area give away large jars of grape jelly with the purchase of peanut butter, so there was certainly no economic incentive for this crazy idea.

I love the taste of seedless grapes, but the only varieties of grapes suitable for home vineyards that flourish in my growing zone have very thick, almost unpalatable, tough skins and are loaded with big seeds. The pulp from these grapes tastes good, but the seedless varieties from California and other places are better tasting to me, are less expensive to buy, and are much easier to eat. Nevertheless, I pursued this vineyard idea for no apparent reason.

My first order of business was to decide what varieties to plant. I remembered from my childhood that my paternal grandparents had several vines of Concord and Niagara grapes in a sunny pasture behind their barn. The reason I knew they were these varieties was because my father told me. As a youngster, they were fun to pick and good to eat in late summer when I visited their subsistence farm, around forty-five miles north of where I now live. As I read more about attempts to locally grow these two varieties, I discovered that they grow better in cooler climates and would likely die after a few years due to the hot summers and a certain vine-destroying insect we have down south. Nevertheless, my logic was that if my grandfather could grow them, why couldn't I? Also, two-year-old specimens were readily available at local nurseries, and why would a nursery sell something that was unsuited for the local climate? So, it was easy to decide to plant these two varieties.

Another variety planted was muscadines. These grapes are native to the southeastern states and grow in two colors—deep purple (often referred to as black) and bronze. Uncultured varieties can be found growing wild in southern woods. When fully ripe, they have a sweet, musky taste, similar to Concords. Cultured varieties produce much larger grapes and are substantially more prolific than those growing wild. In the South, it is common to see muscadine vines growing in home and commercial vineyards.

Like Concords and Niagaras, muscadine grapes are slip-skin and have multiple seeds in them. Eating a slip-skin grape is quite different than a non-slip-skin. The grape is placed between one's thumb and index finger while simultaneously holding the stem side of the fruit between the lips, making an air-tight seal. The grape is sharply squeezed until the skin breaks and the pulp slips into your mouth. Afterward, some people place the skin in their mouths and chew on it slightly to extract the residual pulp. Others have learned to maintain the air-tight seal, described above, as they squeeze harder and suck the residual goodness out. After manipulating the pulp with one's tongue and teeth to separate it from the seeds, the seeds and skins, if chewed, are spit on the ground or disposed of using some less conspicuous method for those who are more culturally refined.

Many varieties of muscadines grow to be much larger than Concords and Niagaras; some are larger in circumference than a quarter. Also, many muscadine cultivars ripen at inconsistent times and grow in small clusters. To harvest most varieties, each grape is picked individually as it ripens instead of gathering the whole cluster. Harvesting a vine from the time ripening begins until all fruit is picked is approximately four to six weeks.

I planted eight Concord, two Niagara, plus four purple and three bronze muscadine vines—seventeen vines total. I learned to train, fertilize, spray, and prune the vines from internet research and talking with my local County Extension Service. After planting, the vines had to grow and develop three years before any grapes could be harvested. If blooms formed prior to the third year, they were pinched off. All energy was necessary for plant development.

I couldn't wait and cheated a little the second year by letting a few of the blooms remain to develop into grapes. There were enough to tease me for what was to happen in future years. That same year, the Niagaras became anemic-looking, and it became apparent that they were not going to produce. By the fourth year, they were dead. Also, one of the bronze muscadine vines remained very thin, and it did not make it. I believe it failed due to being planted in a location with inadequate sun.

By the third year, production was good, but in the fourth through sixth years, it was unbelievable! I truly questioned my sanity for planting all those grapes. There was no way I could possibly use the whole crop—both Concords and muscadines. My guess is that a total of sixty or more gallons of grapes were harvested in each of those years. From mid-July through the end of September, I became a slave to the vineyard. Needless to say I could use only a fraction of the total crop, and I ended up giving most of the grapes away.

I tried to make juice, jam, and jelly but soon discovered that my skill level and equipment were severely inadequate. Some jelly and juice recipes said to stir and press the grapes with a potato masher while they simmered over low heat. Following that, the grapes were to be strained through a finely meshed strainer or cheesecloth. Seeds and skins were discarded. This was supposed to yield juice that could be canned, frozen, or used to make jelly. I tried this method, but the process was incredibly slow and cumbersome; yield was poor; and the juice was cloudy. I discovered that after canning, both the juice and jelly would turn from a purplish-blue to a brownish color by eight months—not very appetizing. The exception was to make jelly with enormous amounts of sugar and boil the solution down until it thickened.

Another method I later tried was to simmer the grapes as described above. But instead of attempting to strain them, I let them cool slightly, and then ground them with an emersion blender while still in the pot. After that, I would run this concoction through a food mill to extract the seeds. This procedure yielded a mushy, thick liquid that I used to make jam—not jelly. I called it jam because, except for the seeds, it contained the whole grape, although in mush form. It was still cloudy, which I knew would be the case. Good jelly is clear.

By now, I had learned to use pectin in the jam recipe, which greatly reduced the amount of required sugar and cook time. I also could use a sugar substitute with the correct type of pectin. I read that citric or ascorbic acid could be added to prevent the jam from turning brown. I got the pectin to work, but, even with added acid, the jam still became discolored after several months.

I knew there was a better way, but it was yet to be found. Finally, I saw a video on YouTube where an extension service representative was making grape juice with a steam juicer. As its name implies, this device uses steam to extract the juice.

The juicer consists of three tiers of pans. The lower tier looks like a small stockpot where water is boiled and steam is generated.

The second tier has an appearance similar to that of a Bundt cake pan but with straight and nondecorative walls; it sits on the boiler pan. One of its purposes is to transfer steam to the top tier through its center cylinder. It also serves as a juice collector and has a tube with a spout that is mounted near its bottom and on its outer wall. A hole is drilled on the lower side of the outer wall, where the tube is attached. This tube provides an exit or siphon path for the juice.

The third and top tier is also a large stockpot-looking

pan with a lid. Its base has numerous small holes drilled in it, similar to a colander. It sits atop the second-tier pan and holds several quarts of raw grapes. As steam is released, it is channeled upward through the cylinder of the middle pan to the top tier, where the grapes are placed. When the steam hits the grapes, they become hot and swell, their skins split, and juice is released. As it is released, it falls through the small holes into the second-tier pan, where it is collected and channeled through the exit tube into a collection vessel, such as a quart mason jar. The result is clear juice with good yield. The skins and seeds remain in the top pan.

After seeing this device, I found one I liked online and ordered it. It worked as advertised. After making the juice, the skins and seeds were discarded. I now had good, transparent juice that I could drink or use to make clear, good-tasting, low-sugar jelly that did not discolor as badly.

In the eighth year, the Concord grape vines started to die, and they were all dead by year eleven, except part of one arm on one vine. It is now year thirteen since planting, and I expect that arm to die soon. The trained horticulturalists were correct. Concord grapes do not grow well in the South. However, the muscadines continue to outdo themselves, yielding between twenty-five and thirty gallons of grapes annually.

4

THE EXPERIMENTAL DIET

Several months before my disappointing PSA result in April 2014, I read from several reliable sources that there was a link between diet and prostate health. I did not give that connection much thought until it became apparent that androgen deprivation therapy was likely on the horizon. After the April report, I began doing extensive research on foods that could potentially slow prostate cancer progression. In doing this research, it was discovered that studies had been performed on laboratory animals and sometimes humans using individual types of foods, some with promising results.

A study that integrated all involved foods and dietary supplements in the diet of actual prostate cancer patients could not be found. I was curious and questioned what the outcome would be if all involved foods were included. It was then that I felt impressed to do an experiment by deliberately integrating as many cancer-fighting foods into my diet as I could.

To begin this self-appointed initiative, the first item that needed to be determined was which foods and dietary supplements to use. For this, the internet was my primary research tool. Although scores of sites were reviewed, many were eliminated. They either turned out to be advertisements or were from what I believed to be unreliable sources. Attention was given to sites that appeared to be legitimate.

Results or reviews of studies performed by one organization were compared against those of another, if two on the same food item could be found. If studies came to no definitive conclusion concerning a particular food or if results were contradictory, that item was usually included in my experiment. Flaxseed and cruciferous vegetables were two examples.

It was discovered that professional opinions varied widely on whether some foods or dietary supplements had a positive, negative, or neutral impact on prostate cancer. Vitamin E was one such example. Some argued that increased use of this vitamin could actually increase the probability of getting prostate cancer, while others argued that it may slow its progression or aid in preventing the disease. Where there were arguments that a food or dietary supplement, such as vitamin E, could potentially cause or increase disease progression, that item was also included, but used with cautious moderation.

The dietary experiment was done in three phases. The first phase was subjective and was not a self-generated or a proactive initiative. Between the time of my radiation and the Mayo Clinic visit, my urologist suggested that I drink pomegranate juice and take a nonprescription nutritional supplement called Prostate 2.4. This nonprescription product is manufactured by a company named Theralogix and can be ordered online. Apparently, it is not on store shelves. It comes in capsule form and contains several vitamins (including vitamin E) and other ingredients that benefit prostate health. I did comply with his recommendations, but it is unknown what impact, if any, these two items made on PSA results. My PSA reading continued to increase, but that increase could have been at a slower rate than it would have been without these products, or it could have been that inadequate time was given for the two products to make an impact.

Phase 2 was started in May 2014, after the April PSA score of 2.73 and after research was finished on which foods to include. This phase ended four months later on August 8, when the result from my next PSA test was known.

Below are foods and dietary supplements that were included in Phase 2. Each item is listed followed with a brief explanation of how that item may impact prostate cancer. Conclusions for each were done after analyzing multiple internet articles and study reviews. Additional personal research can be accomplished by simply entering into an internet browser such things as "foods for prostate cancer" or "prostate cancer and flaxseed" as examples. Note that some items may show different conclusions from different reviews. As stated earlier, only those that appeared to be from unbiased and reliable sources were considered.

Prostate 2.4: Addressed in Phase 1. Information on this product is limited, but some can be obtained from its manufacturer, Theralogix Nutritional Science.

Pomegranate Juice: Several studies show evidence

that long-term consumption of this juice may slow the progression of prostate cancer.

Flaxseed (Not Flax Oil): Flaxseed contain lignans, a compound thought to slow the aggressiveness of prostate cancer. Lignans are also in sesame seeds, pumpkin seeds, and rye. Flax oil was avoided. It appears that flax oil may actually make prostate cancer worse. In the refining process to make oil, lignans remain in the seed but are not present in the oil. Although intake of flaxseed was included in Phase 2, their use was very limited in that no suitable way to integrate them in my diet was found. This changed in Phase 3.

Cruciferous Vegetables: Common cruciferous vegetables include cabbage, brussels sprouts, broccoli, cauliflower, kale, collards, horseradish, turnips, and others. Several studies support the notion that these vegetables may prevent or slow the progression of prostate cancer, but others find no such evidence.

Walnuts: Studies showed that walnuts may slow the progression of prostate cancer in laboratory animals (mice). No studies on humans were found, but it is believed that walnuts (and other nuts) do have medicinal properties.

Tomatoes: Results were inconclusive concerning the impact of tomato consumption on prostate cancer prevention and progression. There was some evidence that eating condensed tomatoes several times weekly slowed cancer growth, but it was far from conclusive, with more study required. Tomatoes as well as red bell peppers and red watermelon contain the antioxidant lycopene.

Fatty Fish: Studies were contradictory as to the benefit of eating fatty fish such as salmon, trout, herring, and mackerel. There appeared to be more evidence that these types of fish were beneficial than against. Some studies found that fatty omega-3 might actually cause prostate cancer.

Resveratrol: This agent is found in the skins of dark-skinned grapes (but possibly not muscadine grapes—studies were contradictory), red wine, and peanuts. It is also available as a dietary supplement and can be purchased in capsule form at big-box stores, pharmacies, health-food stores, and online. This was used in the form of a dietary supplement in my experiment. There is evidence that resveratrol may aid in preventing prostate cancer occurrence and growth, but more study and research is needed to fully support this possibility. Some do not agree that resveratrol, per se, impacts prostate cancer. Rather, they argue that the effect is caused by other agents found in foods from which resveratrol is taken.

Dark Chocolate: Some studies show that dark chocolate may slow cancer progression and have other health benefits. Results from reliable studies were difficult to find.

Research showed that there were other foods that may aid in slowing or preventing prostate cancer, but they were not deliberately included in this experiment. These foods were green tea, soy, vitamin E (included in Prostate 2.4 capsule), tofu, legumes, garlic, blueberries, and others. One recent study showed foods with selenium slowed prostate cancer growth. Selenium is found in certain animal and seafood proteins as well as some vegetables, such as mushrooms. Except for green tea, soy, and tofu, my normal diet included these other foods.

In addition to foods that enhanced prostate health or slowed prostate cancer growth, there were foods to be avoided, such as red meat, charred foods, and high-fat dairy products. Intake of red meat was limited to no more than ten ounces per week (usually less) and exclusive consumption of skim milk and low-fat cheese.

After consuming the above foods for several months, I entered the office of my urologist on August 8, 2014. I was mentally prepared and was expecting to be placed on ADT. Based on recent PSA velocity, this was the time I would likely reach the 5.0 threshold. After waiting in the examining room for a few long and anxious minutes, my doctor entered the room with a smile and said my PSA had stabilized and had declined slightly. It was now 2.45—down from 2.73. What a relief! Perhaps this diet was working. He told me to come back in six months. That visit ended Phase 2 of my experiment. It was now time for Phase 3.

5

THE MIRACLE PUNCH

There was one additional food that laboratory tests showed could potentially kill prostate cancer cells in humans that was not included in Phase 2. It was emerging with great promise, and no studies discrediting initial laboratory work were found. What was this food? *Muscadine skins!* The purpose for all those muscadine grapes was now known. Skins from dark-colored muscadines contain properties other than resveratrol that apparently kill prostate cancer cells but not good cells.

It was now August 2014, and that year's crop of muscadines from my small vineyard was beginning to mature; timing could not have been better. By mid-August, I had enough to make juice. The juice was canned, as usual, but this time the skins were saved. They were partially cooked already from the juicer, but some remained too tough to process. I simmered them in a large stainless-steel soup pot until soft—around twenty minutes. This purple mush-like product was run through my food mill the same way that was used in the jam-making attempt. This separated the skins from the seeds. I now had a muscadine skin paste that I could use for Phase 3 of my experiment, but how could this sticky mush be integrated into my diet? Skins not immediately used were preserved by freezing. These would be thawed and used as needed.

After experimenting, the idea came to use the skins in a punch. To make this punch, I used a high-speed stand blender to mix the muscadine skins with muscadine or grape juice, an artificial sweetener, and flaxseed. Later I began adding green tea leaves. The result was a thick, purplish-pink base that I next mixed with pomegranate juice. This drink was taken with meals, to wash down other pills such as Prostate 2.4 and resveratrol, or consumed by itself. Later, I discovered that a better-tasting drink could be made by adding a small amount of diet ginger ale or sparkling water. With this punch, I was now taking three to six cancer-fighting foods at once: flaxseed, pomegranate juice, muscadine skins, Prostate 2.4, green tea, and resveratrol. I continued to take foods from Phases 1 and 2 while concurrently doing Phase 3.

My next PSA test was scheduled for early February 2015—six months after my previous appointment. Blood was drawn on February 3, and test results were given one week later on February 9. As I anticipated this appointment, my level of anxiety was more intense than usual. I had received an encouraging report six months earlier. Was the result from that test an anomaly? Would my PSA continue to drop, remain stable, or increase? Once again, the doctor was smiling when he entered the room, indicating to me that he was happy. When I saw the report, I was stunned. My PSA had dropped to .46. I couldn't believe it, nor could my doctor. It had dropped so much that he asked me if I had been taking hormones (i.e., ADT) and ordered a second test, which confirmed the .46 reading.

It continued to drop even more at each subsequent six-month test. On Tuesday, August 2, 2016, I received the results from my regular six-month PSA test. My urologist is experienced, probably in his late-fifties or early sixties. No doubt, he has treated all kinds of illnesses and hundreds, maybe thousands, of prostate cancer patients during his career. When he shared the result of this PSA test, he said he had never seen anything like it. Why? *My PSA result was undetectable, accomplished without normal prostate cancer treatment!*

Has this disease been defeated? It is unknown. I am continuing my cancer-fighting diet as well as seeing my doctor. What is known is that at one point the disease had invaded my pelvic lymph nodes (possibly more), was aggressively growing based on velocity of PSA results, had begun to metastasize, was possibly stage IV, and had not been cured with two surgeries and radiation treatment. It is also known that one PSA test was undetectable and one year later (August 2017) was only 0.1, indicating strong disease reversal and possibly complete healing.

6

THE REVELATIONS

Early on Wednesday morning, August 3, 2016, the day following the news that my PSA was undetectable and as I was having my daily private time with the Lord, He revealed to me in a clear and remarkable way several things about my disease reversal. They were items that would likely have never have entered my mind. They hit me like a lightning bolt—one of the strongest revelations from the divine I have ever had!

On that morning, the Holy Spirit (explained below) began revealing to me how He had placed a multitude of seemingly unrelated things in my life over a period of years to make my healing possible. Specifically, it was He who instructed me to plant the vineyard and to try the experimental diet. It was He who had provided the tools, raw materials, and knowledge that was necessary to make the cancer-fighting punch. At the time they happened, they appeared to just be part of daily living with no unusual significance. As the Holy Spirit spoke to me, He revealed how He had directed me and had provided these things for a specific purpose—my healing. Individually, they may appear trivial and coincidental. Collectively, they are part of a well devised and orchestrated plan and an indication of how the Holy Spirit sometimes works. They demonstrate the care God gives to His people, often in very unusual ways.

The Holy Spirit is God's spirit, which is placed in a Christian when that person is forgiven of his or her sins (i.e., born again). The Holy Spirit is the third person of the Holy Trinity—Father, Son, and Holy Spirit. While the Father (God) and Son (Jesus Christ) reside in heaven, the Holy Spirit resides on earth—specifically, in the hearts of Christians. The Holy Spirit speaks to Christians through their consciences. All humans have a sense of right and wrong that provides to them a basic moral code. The Holy Spirit is a gift from God that refines this code but, more importantly, provides direction for one's life that, if obeyed, keeps it consistent with the will and purpose of God.

The Holy Spirit speaks to Christians in several different ways but primarily through the Bible and personal communion (i.e., prayer and meditation). He may also speak through other people, such as a pastor or Bible teacher, a thought, past experiences, literature, poetry, music and art, feelings, notions, His creation, dreams, and others. The Holy Spirit will never direct a person in a way that is contradictory to biblical teachings. Sometimes the Holy Spirit provides strong and clear direction; other times it may be subtle and a whisper. In either case, the Christian should obey that voice, regardless of the way delivered or the circumstance.

In my case, the Holy Spirit was directing me without me even realizing He was speaking. Other Christians may share this same spiritual infirmity. Our minds are often focused more on the horizontal events in our lives (human and earthly things) rather than the vertical (godly and divine) things. Because of this, we don't hear His voice when He speaks. Nevertheless, God and the Holy Spirit still embrace believers when they fail spiritually or when they don't recognize His voice. In Christian circles, this is sometimes referred to as providential care.

Below are the stories behind the acquisition of several pieces of equipment that were needed to make the muscadine punch as well as other significant happenings related to my story. I am convinced that all these items and events were part of God's master plan to allow my life to be extended and, hopefully, the lives of many others. Of all the men in the world suffering from prostate cancer, I am overwhelmed, confused, humbled, and grateful that He allowed this to happen to me. When God performs a miracle, He has a reason.

▌FOOD MILL

The healing process began decades before this story begins, estimated to be in the 1950s or 1960s, when my father-in-law purchased a food mill. My wife has no idea why he bought this piece of equipment. It was never used by him, his wife, or anyone else. After he and my mother-in-law passed away and as the family was disposing of their belongings, the only thing my wife kept without emotional value was this food mill. She had no reason to keep it; she just did. It sat unused in the closet of a spare bedroom in our home until I started experimenting with it when trying to make muscadine jam—some fifty to sixty years after being purchased. This tool turned out to be a valuable asset in separating muscadine seeds from skins. This particular style of food mill, apparently, is no longer available in stores and has to be ordered online. Similar products are manufactured (I bought one) but are not as efficient for my application as this particular design. God provided this simple piece of equipment in an unusual way. I would never have thought to use a food mill had this one not already been available.

VINEYARD

Next is the planting of the muscadine vines. As stated previously, I had no clue at the time why those vines were planted. They were planted on a notion that turned out to be the leading of the Holy Spirit. I did not at all connect my small vineyard at the time of planting with having any medicinal value or use and certainly no spiritual relevance. From my perspective, it was just a new hobby and undertaking. To God, it was a gift to me for my survival.

STEAM JUICER

The steam juicer has a story of its own. I spent days, maybe weeks, over a period of several months trying to find a juicer that would serve my need. Every design I considered had something wrong with it. It was either too expensive, inadequate for the job, or delivered undesired results. At the time, I was not interested in one that would save the skins, but was seeking one that would yield juice. Finally, based on what I perceived to be an accidental find, a steam juicer was demonstrated on a YouTube video that was exactly what I was seeking. Before seeing this design, I had decided to purchase a much more expensive and less efficient device—similar to one used for pressing grapes for wine. The steam juicer delivered good juice and was reasonably priced. This occurred years before I learned of any connection between muscadine skins and their impact on prostate health and cancer.

The remarkable thing about this juicer is that it yielded good juice and saved the skins. Now, its primary use is a tool to deliver muscadine skins while juicing is secondary.

Discovering this product was not by accident, as originally believed, but was by the grace of God. It was through His foreknowledge and the working of the Holy Spirit that directed me to the obscure YouTube video where this product was demonstrated.

PROPANE STOVE

The propane stove was not mentioned in my story but has significance. The kitchen stove in my home is electric with a microwave oven above it. I often plant a small vegetable garden and have a couple of fruit trees as well as the muscadine vines. In the summer I will, occasionally, can certain vegetables and make pickles, sauces, jellies, jams, and preserves. To properly sterilize the glass jars before canning and to kill any bacteria in the food, it is necessary to use a boiling water bath or a pressurized canner, depending on what is being preserved.

Steam from jar sterilization and canning causes the controls on the microwave oven to become wet and dysfunctional. When the controls dry, the microwave once again works, usually after three weeks or so. To prevent this from happening, it was necessary to get another source of heat for canning, which ended up being a free-standing two-burner propane camp stove.

This stove is on four removable legs and, when used, is placed just inside the open basement boat door of my home while the portable propane tank sits barely outside. There is a flexible gas line that connects the two, similar to that on a gas grill. The steam juicer requires a good heat source and generates a lot of steam. The propane stove, while purchased for a different reason, now serves as the source of heat for the juicer. Was this coincidental? It is difficult to determine, but based on other events associated with this story, I believe God provided it for this purpose in a roundabout way.

HIGH-SPEED BLENDER

Next is the story of the high-speed blender. My desire for a high-speed blender did not come from an ad, an immediate need, or infomercial. Instead, it came from a Sunday school class. In this class, it was customary at the time for someone to bring, on a rotational basis, some form of refreshment. Typically, it was sweet rolls, donuts, cookies, and so forth. One Sunday morning, it was the turn of a lady who had just purchased a popular high-speed blender, for which she was very grateful. She wanted to use it for God's work and for other people; that was her nature. She lugged that heavy blender and supplies into the building and placed them on a table in a hallway near the classroom. With them she made something healthy—a smoothie—for everyone in the class. It consisted of several ingredients that only she knows. I know it included kale and blueberries plus other unknown ingredients.

After class she encouraged me to consider buying one to make healthy smoothies. I did give it some thought, but my thinking was not necessarily focused on healthy smoothies but more on smooth milkshakes.

It didn't take long to dismiss the idea of getting one after I discovered what they cost. There was no milkshake or smoothie on earth that was worth that much money! How many trips to the neighborhood ice-cream shop or even a salad bar could I make for the equivalent amount of money?

When I received my next credit card statement, the idea of getting one of these very expensive blenders again occurred to me. I did a bit of investigation and discovered that my account held just enough accumulated points to buy this type of machine. After discussing this matter with my wife and coming to a mutual agreement, we ordered one with the idea of making healthy smoothies. To date, I believe one could count on a single hand the number of smoothies and milkshakes combined the machine has made. However, this device has become a necessity when mixing muscadine skins, flaxseed, sweetener, green tea leaves, and juice as the base for the cancer-fighting punch. It is also used to make almond butter, which is believed by some to slow prostate cancer progression.

This high-speed blender is a tool that is essential for this experimental diet that I am on. Once again, I cannot believe that the circumstances leading to the acquisition of this machine were coincidental. They had to be through the workings of the Holy Spirit. Essentially, the blender was free, purchased with credit card points.

QUANTITIES OF INGREDIENTS

The next extraordinary happening in this series of Spirit-led events was the determination of quantities of foods and dietary supplements to use. I knew nothing about the chemical or nutritional makeup of involved foods nor had any idea concerning what quantity of each to take. My research revealed very little about how much of what to use. It simply exposed that certain foods might help slow, stop, or prevent prostate cancer. The two exceptions were the Prostate 2.4 supplement, which came with instructions to take two capsules daily. The other exception was an article that recommended eight ounces of pomegranate juice daily. As I was trying to resolve this situation, quantities needed and frequency of use started making themselves clear to me. I am almost embarrassed to say that at the time, I did not recognize this revelation as the Holy Spirit speaking but attributed it to logic and reason. That changed with the strong revelation I experienced on August 3. Sometimes God gives us expertise far beyond our levels of skill and knowledge.

KNOWLEDGE FROM FAILURE

While I experienced failure in my initial attempts to make muscadine juice, jam, and jelly, these failures taught me exactly how and what to do to separate muscadine seeds from their skins. This process is necessary when making the cancer-fighting punch. The Holy Spirit allowed me to experience short-term failure in exchange for long-term success.

Many in Christian circles sometimes use the expression, *God works in mysterious ways*. Although this phrase cannot be found as a direct quote from the Bible, based on experience and stories from the Bible, it is a known truth. It is not our human responsibility to know or to understand how God works. We are human, and God is God. It is our responsibility to know God; have a relationship with Him; share Him with others; obey when He speaks; communicate with Him through prayer, Bible study, and meditation; do good works; love everyone, and let Him do His work as only He can.

The prayer of my pastor for my healing was, indeed, answered, but in a completely different way than was expected. Although his prayer seemed to go unanswered at the time from all human measurements and observations, God had already begun answering this prayer many years before it was offered with no one knowing what was going on behind the scenes. It was answered in such a way that has the potential to help many prostate cancer patients prolong their lives.

Humans have dimensional and finite understanding while the workings of God are nondimensional and infinite. Whatever our situations and circumstances, God knows what is best for us. I thank and praise Him daily.

7

THE REVEALED PROSTATE CANCER DIET

If you have prostate cancer and are considering going on all or parts of this diet, it is suggested that you discuss it first with your doctor. It could potentially interact with medications you are taking or cause other adverse reactions due to allergies. Some of the foods are high in sugar and potassium; the diet also contains nuts. Therefore, it may not be suitable for some diabetics, those with high potassium levels, those with nut allergies, or other conditions. Again, discuss with your doctor. Be forewarned that he or she may be suspicious of the effectiveness of the diet.

Please understand that this combination of foods and supplements seems to be working wonders for me, but it may not work for all. Therefore, I can only be accountable for their effect on me, and they should be used by you solely at your own discretion. Consuming these foods is in no way intended to be used as a substitute for normal professional care and medical advice.

You may be asking at what point in disease progression these foods should be consumed. My personal strategy is to use them during watchful waiting periods. Prostate cancer, in many cases, is slow growing, and a doctor may recommend deferring surgery, radiation, or other treatments until the disease has reached some threshold. It is during these waiting periods that the diet could potentially be most effective. If your body responds, it could defer your next line of defense for many years or even permanently. To date, it has postponed my next set of treatments (i.e., ADT) for over three years. Every six months I have a routine PSA test to ensure the disease is under control. I may never have to go to the next step if the diet continues to work. But if I do, I will likely suspend the diet during treatments. My reasoning is that it could affect the results of medical treatment. When treatments are completed, it will be resumed. Please view this diet as complementary to normal medical care.

The diet has become a personal lifestyle and is easy. Most of it is healthy as well as tasty. It is not inexpensive, but it is financially manageable.

THE PROSTATE CANCER DIET

- Two Prostate 2.4 capsules daily: one with breakfast and the other at dinner.

- One serving of cruciferous vegetables daily, broccoli preferred.

- One ounce of walnuts daily.

- 250mg of Resveratrol daily. I take mine in the morning as a dietary supplement.

- Five-eighths ounce of dark chocolate (at least 60 percent cacao) daily.

- Two to three servings of fatty fish weekly (salmon, trout, mackerel, herring, albacore tuna). Note: I eat trout and salmon exclusively. Other types of fresh fatty fish are not readily available in my area.

- Two servings of condensed tomatoes weekly. Examples of use are marinara sauce, tomato-basil soup, and other tomato-based soups and stews. Fresh tomatoes, although delicious and healthy, don't provide many cancer-fighting properties. Red bell pepper and red watermelon also contain cancer-fighting properties.

- No more than ten ounces of red meat weekly, limited char-cooked foods, no high-fat dairy products.

- Ten to twelve ounces of muscadine skin punch daily. Recipe follows. I typically drink two and a half to three ounces in the morning, five to six ounces with lunch (I add around three ounces of diet ginger ale to mine at lunch), and two and a half to three ounces in the evenings.

- Maintain a positive mental attitude. It can be argued that a positive attitude coupled with hopeful expectation can and do impact end results.

RECIPE FOR MUSCADINE SKIN PUNCH

Note: Making this punch is a two-step process. First, a concentrated mixer is made. Second, the concentrate is mixed with pomegranate juice.

1. Recipe for the Mixer
   - 1 cup muscadine skin paste/mush
   - 2/3 cup ground flax seed
   - 3 to 4 tablespoons sweetener of your choice to taste (optional—muscadine skins aren't sweet)
   - 1 quart of muscadine juice or dark grape juice
   - 4 tablespoons bulk green tea leaves

Place all the above ingredients in a high-speed blender and blend on high for at least ninety seconds. Yield is approximately 1 1/4 quarts. Keep refrigerated. One batch of mixer lasts two weeks.

2. Blending Mixer with Pomegranate Juice
   - 1 cup plus 1 tablespoon muscadine skin mixer
   - 3 cups pomegranate juice (I use the type in the chilled juice section of the supermarket rather than the bottled variety, due to better taste.)

Place juice and mixer in container, such as an empty milk jug, and shake well initially and again before each use.

Keep refrigerated.

Drink nine to ten ounces daily. Hint: It is easier to blend a double recipe, which lasts approximately one week.

An issue with this diet is finding a source for muscadine skins. However, muscadine skin extract (MSKE) is available online and is sold as a dietary supplement. I have not tried it and cannot confirm or deny its effectiveness nor recommend how much to use.

MSKE was used instead of actual skins in research studies with positive results. If it is used, perhaps replacing the muscadine skins with MSKE would work. MSKE is sold in both powder and capsule form. If MSKE is used, take it as recommended from the supplier or manufacturer. In addition, blend for sixty seconds on high speed 1/3 cup of ground flaxseed, 1 3/4 quarts pomegranate juice, and 2 tablespoons bulk green tea leaves. Drink eight ounces per day. No sweetener should be needed with this combination in that pomegranate juice is very sweet. If MSKE works as well as actual muscadine skins, using it would certainly require less effort, would be more easily sourced, and likely less expensive.

If you are suffering from prostate cancer or a rising PSA, my prayer is that you will have complete healing. If you choose to use the above diet, my hope is that it will work as well for you as it is for me.

May God bless you, give you peace and good health, and may His richest blessings be bestowed on you!

Printed in the United States
By Bookmasters